HIGH BLOOD PRESSURE

THINGS YOU SHOULD KNOW
(QUESTIONS AND ANSWERS)

By Rumi Michael Leigh

Introduction

I would like to thank and congratulate you for downloading this book, " *High Blood Pressure, things you should know (questions and answers)*" series.

This book will help you understand, revise and have a good general knowledge and keywords of high blood pressure and how it affects the lives of people who suffer from high blood pressure.

Thanks again for downloading this book, I hope you enjoy it!

Chapter 1

1) What is hypertension?

- Hypertension is the increase in blood pressure due to the narrowing of arteries.

2) What is another name for hypertension?

- Another name for hypertension is high blood pressure.

3) What is the value of normal blood pressure?

- The normal value of blood pressure is 120/80.

4) What does 120 represent in normal blood pressure?

- 120 represents the heart's contraction.

5) What does 80 represent in normal blood pressure?

- 80 represents the heart's relaxation.

6) Why is hypertension considered a silent killer?

- Hypertension is considered a silent killer because a person can have hypertension for a longtime without knowing and it usually doesn't present any symptoms.

7) What are the causes of hypertension?

- The causes of hypertension are stress, high cholesterol, obesity, smoking, excessive caffeine consumption, family history, lack of physical activity, age, diabetes, pregnancy, chronic kidney disease, etc.

8) How is blood pressure measured?

- Blood pressure is measured by using a sphygmomanometer.

9) What does blood pressure depend on?

- Blood pressure depends on cardiac output and systemic arterial resistance.

Chapter 2

1) Is exercise dangerous for people with high blood pressure?

- No, exercise is not dangerous for people with high blood pressure. People with high blood pressure should exercise moderately.

2) How can blood pressure be lowered?

- Blood pressure can be lowered by physical exercises, by stopping smoking, by weight loss, by decrease in alcohol, a healthy diet (and a decrease in salt consumption), etc.

3) How long is the treatment of high blood pressure?

- High blood pressure is treated for life.

4) Name the common precautionary signs of hypertension.

- The common precautionary signs of hypertension are bleeding from the nose, headaches, etc.

5) What are the goals of antihypertensive therapy?

- The goals of antihypertensive therapy are to normalize arterial pressure and prevent complications.

6) Define vasoconstriction.

- Vasoconstriction is the narrowing of blood vessels.

7) What is the effect of vasoconstriction?

- The effect of vasoconstriction is the increase in blood pressure.

8) Define vasodilation.

- Vasodilation is the widening of blood vessels.

9) What is the effect of vasodilation?

- The effect of vasodilation is the decrease in blood pressure.

10) What are the dangers of processed food in relation to hypertension?

- The dangers of processed food in relation to hypertension is that processed food contains a lot of salt that contributes to hypertension.

Chapter 3

1) What is prehypertension?

- Prehypertension is the first stage of high blood pressure. It is when the value of blood pressure is slightly or moderately higher than normal. It is a warning sign.

2) What is malignant hypertension?

- Malignant hypertension is a very high blood pressure and a medical emergency.

3) What is a major danger of malignant hypertension?

- A major danger of malignant hypertension is that it can cause organ damage.

4) What are the main types of hypertension?

- The main types of hypertension are primary and secondary hypertension.

5) What is primary hypertension?

- Primary hypertension is a high blood pressure that develops gradually over a very long time without any specific cause.

6) What is another name for primary hypertension?

- Another name for primary hypertension is essential hypertension.

7) What is secondary hypertension?

- Secondary hypertension is high blood pressure that appears suddenly due to health diseases or conditions such as congenital, kidney diseases, etc.

8) Name the diseases caused by high blood pressure.

- The diseases caused by high blood pressure are heart failure, coronary insufficiency, stroke, kidney failure, arteritis, rhythm disorder, blindness, etc.

9) What is another name for cardiac infarction?

- Another name for cardiac infarction is a heart attack.

10) Can hypertension affect the brain?

- Yes, hypertension can affect the brain.

Chapter 4

1) How does hypertension affect the brain?

- Hypertension can affect the brain by causing stroke.

2) What is a stroke?

- A stroke is a lack of supply of blood flow to the brain and causes cell death.

3) What are the types of stroke?

- The types of stroke are ischemic and hemorrhagic stroke.

4) What is ischemic stroke?

- Ischemic stroke is a stroke due to a lack of blood flow.

5) What is hemorrhagic stroke?

- Hemorrhagic stroke is a stroke due to bleeding.

6) How does hypertension affect the kidneys?

- Hypertension affects the kidneys by causing kidney failure.

7) What is kidney failure?

-      This is when the kidney can no longer perform its
       function.

8) What is arteritis?

-      Arteritis is when the walls of the arteries become
       inflamed.

9) What is natriuresis?

-      Natriuresis is the urinary elimination of sodium.

10) How does hypertension affect the heart?

-      Hypertension affects the heart by causing
       congestive heart failure.

Chapter 5

1) What medicines are used for the treatment of blood pressure?

- Medicines used for the treatment of high blood pressure include diuretics, calcium channel blockers, beta-blockers, alpha-blockers, antihypertensives, vasodilators, angiotensin-2 receptor antagonists.

2) What are the indications of diuretics?

- The indications of diuretics are the treatment of hypertension, edema, heart failure, etc.

3) What are the classifications of diuretics?

- The classifications of diuretics are loop diuretics, osmotic diuretics, potassium-sparing diuretics and thiazides diuretics.

4) What are the characteristics of loop diuretics?

- The characteristics of loop diuretics are that loop diuretics are fast, powerful and short-lived.

5) What is the duration of loop diuretics?

- The duration of loop diuretics is 6 hours.

6) Give an example of a loop diuretic.

- An example of a loop diuretic is Lasix.

7) What is edema?

- Edema is the accumulation of fluids in a tissue.

8) What are the general side effects of diuretics?

- The general side effects of diuretics are dehydration, thirst, allergy, renal failure, hypotension, hypokalemia, hyponatremia.

9) What are the characteristics of thiazide diuretics?

- The characteristics of thiazide diuretics are medium efficiency and hyperglycemic.

10) Give an example of a thiazide diuretics.

- An example of a thiazide diuretics is Esidrex.

Chapter 6

1) What are the characteristics of potassium-sparing diuretics?

- Potassium-sparing diuretics are slow and cause the loss of potassium.

2) What is the function of potassium to the heart?

- Potassium enables the heart work efficiently.

3) Which diuretics can cause impotence in men?

- Potassium-sparing diuretics can cause impotence in men.

4) What is hyperkalemia?

- Hyperkalemia is a high level of potassium in the blood.

5) What are the signs of hyperkalemia?

- The signs of hyperkalemia are anxiety, abdominal cramps, diarrhea, arrhythmia, etc.

6) What is hypokalemia?

- Hypokalemia is a low level of potassium in the blood.

7) What are the signs of hypokalemia?

\-   The signs of hypokalemia are cramps, tiredness, nausea and vomiting, rhythm disorder.

8) What is natremia?

\-   Natremia is the concentration of sodium in the blood.

9) What is called a high concentration sodium level in the blood?

\-   A high concentration of sodium level in the blood is called hypernatremia.

10) What is called a low concentration sodium level in the blood?

\-   A low concentration of sodium level in the blood is called hyponatremia.

Chapter 7

1) What are the signs of hyponatremia?

- The signs of hyponatremia are muscular weakness, dizziness, cramps.

2) What is the function of angiotensin-converting enzyme inhibitors?

- Angiotensin-converting enzyme inhibitors prevent the conversion of angiotensin 1 to angiotensin 2.

3) What are the contraindications for angiotensin-converting enzyme inhibitors?

- The contraindications for angiotensin-converting enzyme inhibitors are renal failure, hyperkalemia, pregnancy, breastfeeding, etc.

4) What is the function of angiotensin 2?

- Angiotensin 2 is a powerful vasoconstrictor.

5) What are the antagonists of angiotensin 2?

- The antagonists of angiotensin 2 are Sartans.

6) What is the active power of angiotensin 1?

- None, there is no active power of angiotensin 1.

7) What is needed to activate angiotensin 1?

- Angiotensin-converting enzyme is needed to activate angiotensin 1.

8) What is the role of angiotensin-converting enzyme inhibitors in relation to natriuresis?

- The role of angiotensin-converting enzyme inhibitors in relation to natriuresis is that angiotensin-converting enzyme inhibitors cause an increase in natriuresis and induce renal vasodilation.

9) What are the side effects of angiotensin-converting enzyme inhibitors?

- The side effects of angiotensin-converting enzyme inhibitors are dry cough, hyperkalemia, etc.

10) Explain the mechanism of the renin-angiotensin system.

- Renin works with angiotensinogen to produce angiotensin 1 and becomes angiotensin 2 with the presence of a converting enzyme which finally causes vasoconstriction and aldosterone release.

Chapter 8

1) What are the side effects of inhibitor converting enzymes?

- The side effects of inhibitor converting enzymes are hyperkalemia, decreased glomerular filtration, low blood pressure, dry cough, asthenia, etc.

2) What happens when inhibitor converting enzymes are taken with lithium?

- There is an increase in lithemia when inhibitor converting enzymes are taken with lithium.

3) What is lithemia?

- Lithemia is the presence of excess uric acid in the blood.

4) What are the functions of betablockers?

- Betablockers slow down or decrease the workload of the heart.

5) What are the side effects of betablockers?

- The side effects of betablockers are bradycardia, low blood pressure, heart failure, hypoglycemia, asthenia, allergy, impotence, etc.

6) What are the absolute contraindications for betablockers?

- The absolute contraindications for betablockers are asthma and patients who have a pulse less than 50 beats per minute.

7) What are the relative contraindications for betablockers?

- The relative contraindications for betablockers are heart failure, diabetes etc.

8) Can you abruptly stop taking betablockers?

- No, you cannot abruptly stop taking betablockers.

9) How do you stop taking betablockers?

- You stop taking betablockers gradually.

10) What can happen to abrupt discontinuation of betablockers?

- Abrupt discontinuation of betablockers can cause risk of infarction, headache, tremor, cardiac arrest, risk of sudden death, rhythm disorders, etc.

Chapter 9

1) Why do betablockers need to be stopped 24-48 hours before an operation?

- Betablockers need to be stopped 24-48 hours before an operation because of decrease in blood volume.

2) Give an example of a drug class for blood pressure that affects cardiac output.

- Betablockers.

3) What is cardiac output?

- Cardiac output is the number of beats per minute of the heart.

4) What is negative chronotropic?

- Negative chronotropic is a decreased heart rate.

5) What is negative dromotropic?

- Negative dromotropic is a decrease in the speed of atrioventricular conduction.

6) What is positive inotropic?

- Positive inotropic is an increase in the force of contraction of the myocardium.

7) What is myocardium?

- Myocardium is the involuntary muscular tissue of the heart.

8) Can cold medications cause high blood pressure?

- Yes, cold medications can cause high blood pressure.

9) How do cold medications cause high blood pressure?

- Cold medications can cause high blood pressure because they contain NSAIDS.

10) What are NSAIDS?

- NSAIDS are nonsteroidal anti-inflammatory drugs that help relieve pain, decrease inflammation, reduce fever and prevent blood clots.

Chapter 10

1) Can high blood pressure affect the eyes?

- Yes, high blood pressure can affect the eyes.

2) How does high blood pressure affect the eyes?

- High blood pressure can affect the retina and cause blurry vision.

3) Could hypertension lead to dementia?

- Yes, hypertension could lead to dementia.

4) How could hypertension lead to dementia?

- Hypertension could lead to dementia by an insufficient blood flow to the brain due to the narrowing of arteries.

5) What is asthenia?

- Asthenia is weakness or lack of energy of the body. It could be the whole body or some parts of the body.

6) Which diuretics can cause irreversible deafness?

- Loop diuretics can cause irreversible deafness.

7) What are the signs of dehydration?

- The signs of dehydration are thirst, dry mouth, increased skin folds, etc.

8) What are the side effects of Sartans?

- The side effects of Sartans are dizziness, fatigue, hyperkalemia, hypotension, hypoglycemia, renal failure, etc.

9) What are the counter indications of Sartans?

- The counter indications of Sartans are hepatic insufficiency, renal failure, pregnancy.

10) What are the contraindications of anti-calcium medications?

- The contraindications of anti-calcium medications are pregnancy and breastfeeding, hypotension, sinus dysfunction, etc.

Chapter 11

1) What are the effects of calcium channel blockers?

- Calcium channel blockers decrease the force of contraction of the heart, therefore decrease the work of the heart.

2) What are the indications of calcium channel blockers?

- The indications of calcium channel blockers are high blood pressure, heart failure, etc.

3) What are the side effects of calcium channel blockers?

- The side effects of calcium channel blockers are headache, palpitations, constipation, hypotension, edema of the lower extremities, etc.

Conclusion

Thank you again for downloading this book. I hope it has helped you in your journey to understanding high blood pressure and how it affects the people around you who suffer from it.

Please, if you enjoyed this book, I would like you to leave a review. It'd be appreciated.

Thank you.

www.ingramcontent.com/pod-product-compliance
Lightning Source LLC
Chambersburg PA
CBHW031922270726
48655CB00007BA/3231